BEYOND THE DIAGNOSIS: WORLD SEEN THROUGH THE STETHOSCOPE

COMPILED AND EDITED BY DR. SIDDHI SHAH

Contents

Contents

INTRODUCTION

Beyond the Diagnosis: World Seen Through The Stethoscope was conceived from a deep desire to illuminate the stories that resonate beneath the surface of medicine. This book is more than a collection of medical facts; it is a tribute to the human experiences that infuse life into healthcare. Within these pages, we aim to capture the essence of what it truly means to be part of this noble profession—where every stethoscope hears more than just heartbeats, but stories of courage, compassion, and change.

This anthology brings together the voices of 22 dedicated healthcare professionals who share their personal journeys, offering an intimate glimpse into the moments that have shaped their careers. These stories are not merely accounts of success but are filled with the struggles, triumphs, vulnerabilities, and resilience that define the practice of medicine. Through their narratives, we are reminded that behind every diagnosis is a human being—both the patient and the practitioner—each with their own story to tell.

Medicine is often viewed through the lens of science—measurable, precise, and clinical. However, as the stories in this book reveal, medicine is equally an art, rich with empathy, intuition, and an understanding of the human spirit. *Beyond the Diagnosis* weaves a tapestry of narratives that explore this delicate balance between science and humanity, offering readers a deeper understanding of the medical profession.

Prepare to embark on a journey that goes beyond the clinical confines of healthcare. This book is a collection of stories from those who have committed their lives to healing others, often navigating the complexities of their profession with both skill and heart. These narratives capture the authors at critical junctures in their careers, reflecting on experiences that have shaped their paths. Over time, their ongoing achievements and personal growth have only deepened the meaning of these stories, making them even more inspiring and relevant today.

We hope this book serves as a beacon of inspiration for healthcare professionals, students, and anyone interested in the world of medicine. It is our hope that these stories will spark meaningful conversations about patient care, remind us that medicine is as much about humanity as it is about knowledge, and inspire all of us to strive for excellence in our lives. Let us honor those who dedicate their lives to the well-being of others, and let these stories encourage you to make a positive impact in the world. Wherever we come from, and wherever we are headed, it is our stories that define us, and it is through these stories that our legacy will endure.

CHAPTER I

From Classroom Dreams to ICU Triumphs

-By Dr. Siddhi Shah (MBBS, HBTMC and Dr. R.N. Cooper Municipal General Hospital, Mumbai)

Watching the sun dip below Mumbai's skyline, I stood by my local hospital room window in deep contemplation. The bustling city below appeared so far away from the powerful whirlpool of my MBBS ride and internship. It had been a whirlwind of studying through the night, missing meals as I navigated challenges and hit moments that made me learn and grow in new ways.

My Odyssey began from the pulsating core of Mumbai. But by day one of med school, I was set on changing it all. Lectures, clinical rotations and notes were the staples of my days. I clearly remember my first face-to-face encounter with a real-life patient in my third year. That day had been a rain-soaked one - the sort that caused even breathing to feel uncomfortably heavy and as though life was pulling me down with it towards some kind of end, but no more alive for all its slipping. The hospital buzzed with light electric vertebrate beeps and whispers on pull-out page sighs from behind desksqueeze-squeak-dreary. I was posted in the Internal Medicine ward and I came across Mr. Shinde there, an elderly man struggling with a complex mix of diabetes and hypertension.

I walked over to Mr. Shinde's bed, my hands shaking a bit too aggressive than what I intended them to be. I slightly unsure of myself as started the assessment. The family of the patient, distressed and alarmed, watched upon me hopefully. I made clumsy and awkward first attempts to comfort them. She did her very best to reassure him, but felt like anything she said was not cutting it. But, after weeks upon weeks she did find her groove. Then how to listen more intently, empathise for real and communicate a bit better. My mentor, was great at making the complicated cases seem as an opportunity for growth and learning.

Mr. Shinde had one especially difficult day when his situation deteriorated significantly. I was immersed in the heat of a high pressure environment, working side by with my mentor. His vitals were watched closely, important changes were made in his treatment plan and it was a sleepless working hour after another. There was tension in the ward. I never lost hope in my mission...to make Mr. Shinde feel better. I was there with his worried family and spent those hours recognizing the critical care lessons that even now have not ceased to arrive.

The first day of my internship was both exciting and nerve-wracking for. I needed to put all of that knowledge I learned in the classroom into action. She landed in the high-paced world of an emergency department, seeing patients across the whole spectrum from minor complaints through to life-threatening emergencies. Every day was different and required adrenaline rushes, knee-jerk attentiveness and the constant challenge of keeping one's cool.

There was one case, in particular, that I remember when a 65-year-old man with lungs as bad after five days than our COVID-19 patients were at their worst - so we started buying anticoagulants... I was asked to put in a central line, and had mixed emotions of fear and resolve. This is a high stakes situation, the patient in serious condition. My hands were trembling as I prepped for the procedure. The ICU was a flurry of activity, with nurses and doctors scurrying around me.

I felt the pressure of the moment with each step. The tension in the room was still alive, with every eye on me as I did a complicated dance. I moved pursuit of curriculum under the guidance of senior residents whispering support and urging my fingers into methodical whorls. I wiped the sweat ridding my brow-keen eyesight not leaving that space. Then, with a final definitive push, I confidently slid the central line on for my first try. It was such a relief and the family of that patient were incredibly grateful. I immediately had a surge of victory and so much relief. It ended up being an unforgettable moment for me.

In the evenings, I would frequently be in the hospital library analyzing cases and brainstorming about complicated scenarios with my fellow interns. We would go on to be an incredible support system for each other. We used to share our tales, traded tips and celebrated each one of the baby steps together. During difficult moments the connection that we made became an anchor.

I had a night shift I will never forget when we brought in, among others, a young mother and her newborn child who was having difficulty breathing. Time was running out and I had to act fast. With the assistance of one senior resident, I was able to resuscitate that baby and provide some reassurance for its mother. The experience, among many others was emotionally rewarding. The fear, urgency and relief that flooded through me was a challenging mix all nested within the reason I went into medicine in the first place.

As my internship came to an end, it reflected on the long hours of labor, the highs and lows, and all that was learned. I had come a long way from being an apprehensive student to a strong compassion driven doctor willing to take the leap into her next stage of medical life.

Walking out of the hospital for what would hopefully be her last time as an intern, I breathed a sigh of relief and peered down at the cityscape. The colourful lights of Mumbai appeared to mirror my excitement and uneasiness about the future, I had struggled, I had triumphed and most importantly, I was now a strong physician who would take what came to my head on. Armed with a hopeful heart and a head full of knowledge, I had entered the new world - Medicine; all set to face up to its challenges coming my way.

CHAPTER II

Scrubs vs Stereotypes

-By Dr. Antara Agrawal

During my two-month long surgery rotations in final year, I struck up conversations with a few senior women surgeons at my hospital.

The seniormost lady surgeon told me that her partner, whom she had been with since school, would only agree to marry her if she dropped the idea of becoming a surgeon.

Another doctor recounted that when her parents were circulating her biodata in their social circle to get *"rishtas"* for marriage, at least five men rejected the proposal simply because she was training to be a surgeon. She also narrated the story of a former colleague that when she informed her parents about her keen interest in choosing surgery for her postgraduation twenty years back, she was dragged by her family to a saint to force her to change her mind.

These anecdotes are not isolated incidents or a blip in the trend. Women have faced obstacles in the entry, progress, and success in the field of medicine since the dawn of medicine itself. Though medicine has been practiced in India since centuries, our country got its first female doctor of modern medicine in the name of Anandibai Gopalrao Joshi in the 1880s, just a mere century and a half back. [1]

Even today women doctors make up less than 25% of the healthcare workforce. The numbers are even more dismal in the historically male dominated field of surgery, with women surgeons accounting for just about 10% of the surgeons in India.[2]

Even though the gender chasm in medicine is slowly narrowing and now medical schools often have a 50:50 ratio of boys and girls, very few women cross the bridge from an MBBS degree to an MS degree.

It's a steep pyramid, with women getting shed off at every stage, their feet slipping off or being dragged down at every step. While girls enter medical college in almost equal numbers as boys, fewer than a quarter step into the male-dominated halls of surgical residency, with scantier numbers making it out, or climbing the ladders of subspeciality and donning leadership roles.[3]

The reasons behind this attrition in women surgeons date back to how our society traditionally assigns roles to the genders. While men are expected to be breadwinners, women are supposed to take care of home and hearth. In the Indian community, women are not only responsible for household duties and child-rearing but also expected to participate in social rituals traditionally performed by women.[4]

However, the demanding nature of surgical specialities is universal, whether in the West or in India, and aspiring women surgeons are expected to manage both spheres with equal vigour.

With the responsibilities of starting and raising a family, many girls who are keen to take up a surgical branch begin to doubt their inclinations and are deterred from making a decision that will compromise the care of her kin. The system makes female medical graduates gravitate towards branches that provide more "work-life balance" which essentially translates to letting a woman work within the limitations of stringent gender roles that are averse to change and modification.

Women that do battle and balance the home front, face a whole different potpourri of challenges at work. The preexisting bias and deeply entrenched notion by the large fraternity of male surgeons that women are a liability to the field rather than an asset and make subpar surgeons creates a massive hurdle for women to progress and succeed. [2]

There is a general wariness and scepticism not only amongst colleagues but also the patient population of the skillset and clinical acumen of female surgeons. A female surgical resident I spoke with, working in a government hospital, mentioned that she and her female colleagues "often have to work twice as hard to be taken half as seriously" as their male counterparts.

Contrary to prevailing notions, multiple studies have shown that patients treated by female surgeons had better post operative outcomes and were less likely to experience readmissions and complications.[5,6]

This disadvantageous work environment isn't just limited to the discrimination the women face in a largely all-boys' club. Studies have shown that women pursuing surgical careers had experienced sexual harassment and had cited workplace harassment as one of the factors pushing them to leave their training midway.[7,8]

Many young female surgeons express concerns about the lack of women mentors and role models to look up to. The paucity of mentorship has a negative impact in moulding the decisions and career paths of aspiring women surgeons.[9]

Despite all the roadblocks, women still navigate the tricky paths of surgery and are making a name for themselves. Female surgeons are heading departments of many prestigious public as well as private surgical facilities and playing a pivotal role in healthcare policy-making, both clinically and administratively. Promoting and supporting the equal participation of the female surgeon will take a multipronged approach to tackle obvious as well as implicit barriers. As women rise higher in more influential roles, the issue of pay-disparity should be addressed and solved. Mentorship programs to promote girls in surgery must run from the early years of medical college to make sure that no dream dies before it is even dreamt. A more conducive hospital environment must be encouraged to prevent dropouts in training years.

Promoting women doctors doesn't merely fulfil the task of balancing the gender ratio in medicine. Ramanna et al observed that as the number of females doctors burgeoned at the end of the 20th century, so did the populations of female patients.[10] This phenomenon underscores how a woman doesn't just lift herself up but lifts society up with her too. The scalpel may save lives, but a woman wielding a scalpel may enhance them too.

1.Sood M, Chadda R. Women physicians in India. *Natl Med J India.* 2008;21:154.

2.Bashir S. Why Do We Need More Women in Surgery? *Indian J Colo-Rectal Surg.* 2022;5(1):1. doi:10.4103/ijcs.ijcs_3_22

3.Kass RB, Souba WW, Thorndyke LE. Challenges Confronting Female Surgical Leaders: Overcoming the Barriers. *J Surg Res.* 2006;132(2):179-187. doi:10.1016/j.jss.2006.02.009

4.Sagar S. *Women in Surgery- A Perspective from India.*; 2016.

5.Wallis CJD, Jerath A, Aminoltejari K, et al. Surgeon Sex and Long-Term Postoperative Outcomes Among Patients Undergoing Common Surgeries. *JAMA Surg.* 2023;158(11):1185-1194. doi:10.1001/jamasurg.2023.3744

6.Wallis CJ, Ravi B, Coburn N, Nam RK, Detsky AS, Satkunasivam R. Comparison of postoperative outcomes among patients treated by male and female surgeons: a population based matched cohort study. *BMJ.* 2017;359:j4366. doi:10.1136/bmj.j4366

7.Khoushhal Z, Hussain MA, Greco E, et al. Prevalence and Causes of Attrition Among Surgical Residents: A Systematic Review and Meta-analysis. *JAMA Surg.* 2017;152(3):265-272. doi:10.1001/jamasurg.2016.4086

8.Burgos CM, Josephson A. Gender differences in the learning and teaching of surgery: a literature review. *Int J Med Educ.* 2014;5:110-124. doi:10.5116/ijme.5380.ca6b

9.Xepoleas MD, Munabi NCO, Auslander A, Magee WP, Yao CA. The experiences of female surgeons around the world: a scoping review. *Hum Resour Health.* 2020;18(1):80. doi:10.1186/s12960-020-00526-3

10.Khattar S. Women in Modern Medicine in India: Progression, Contribution, Challenges and Empowerment. *Australas Account Bus Finance J.* 2019;13:88-106. doi:10.14453/aabfj.v13i2.6

CHAPTER III

The Oncall Night

-By Dr. Samruddhi Mane (MBBS, GMC Miraj)

Heading back to 2nd June 2023 midnight, or you can say my birthday morning, I experienced the purest form of love in the most difficult time of their life, the bond between my patient Ariba and her mother.

Kids have always been the most cheerful and positive beings around with whom I love spending my time. On this very note I had joined as a House Officer in the Department of Paediatrics of a District Municipal Hospital in Mumbai.

It was 2nd June, a day before my birthday and with the little excitement we have as adults for our birthdays I had exchanged my duty with my colleague which was falling on the very 3rd. Our On-calls are 24hr shift starting from 8AM to 8AM succeeding day. With the day progressing, my ward started flooding with new indoor admissions, particularly because of the start of monsoon and how these tiny tots were now back from their long summer holidays.

Amongst them was a 3yr old wheatish skin, light coloured eye, cheerful Ariba who was admitted to the ward 4 days ago for lobar Pneumonia and was started with all necessary antibiotics and oxygen supplementation via nasal cannula. With every passing day Ariba's dropping oxygen saturation and spreading of consolidation to the other lung called for shifting her from General ward to ICU. My hospital did not have a paediatric ICU and because of the limited resources there was a need for her shifting to a higher centre. Since we did not have a functioning CPAP, my Senior Resident and I made a bubble CPAP out from Burette Infusion set, Three-way cannula, O2 tubing and distilled water. After explaining to the parents, the need for transfer to a higher centre and making them aware of her deteriorating health, they believed she would get better here and denied.

As the day progressed, on ticking of the clock at 12:00AM with my busy duty, I managed to answer calls of my well-wishers. Certainly, in the midst of a silent night, noticing the entire ward is stable with the only sound of a nebulization of a patient, my eyes stopped to Ariba's bed. She was in a propped-up position with an O2 mask which seemingly disturbed her sleep, she simply raised her hands towards her mother calling for a hug. Looking at this her mother dropped in tears and came closer to take her child in her arms, in no time did she realize the dropping saturation which further made her pause and with heavy heart she backed off Ariba. This sight never got out of my memory, and I felt connected to them, for even today cold shivers run throughout my body when I think of it. It was 4AM and after 2 more admissions I took a short nap and asked the nursing staff to inform in case of need.

With the fine rays of Dawn gently filtering through the curtains, a soft glow began to illuminate the room, just like I would have imagined for the start of my birthday. Realizing my duty would get over in a few hours my eyes snap opened. The ward seemed peaceful and calm as I entered, like holding its breath in the anticipation of the day.

It was 8AM, after giving the call out to my relieving colleague, I turned to Ariba's bed to make her mother realize the need for transfer of her child to higher centre. Understanding this, she consented and after the morning rounds of my Seniors and Attendant she was Ambulated to nearest Tertiary Care. I took the mother's contact number which made me feel better. The only thing I wished to do now was go home and give my mother a tight hug.

Couple of days later I contacted Ariba's mother enquiring about her health, I sensed the pain in her voice. she exclaimed the improvement in her health and how Ariba had the need for Intubation and now has been back to nasal prongs to getting better. She expressed her gratitude towards me and the hospital staff. On learning this, I heaved a sigh of Relief and my heart felt lighter.

It was this day again which gave me my purpose and joy of being a doctor and helping others despite of the overwhelming workload, The learning, The empathizing and watching the Process of Healing and the results thereafter always brings Eternal Satisfaction.

CHAPTER IV

The Missing Link

-By Darshak Sanyal and Sharvari Joshi

Her eyes never seemed to meet mine, as she described a problem rather vaguely in her "chest area". I clearly recall interviewing this elderly woman in my 2nd year Surgery rotation, with a large irregular breast mass. She had noticed it several months prior, however out of embarrassment, she was reluctant to report it. By the time she had sought medical attention, it had metastasized widely. At the time, my inexperience prevented me from understanding her point of view. We came from widely different sections of society and her conservatism made no sense to me. I wanted to have played so many roles for her; to have taught her self-breast examinations, educated her about regular screenings, and gently explain that there is no shame in it. But how could I, when she was hesitant to even mention her breasts. There was a missing link that was difficult to overcome.

In a workshop meant to sensitize volunteers on Gender Inclusivity in Healthcare, the presenters sought to invite a few trans individuals to speak about their experiences as patients. However, they refused the invitation and only permitted transcripts of their interviews to be shared with us. They spoke about the disgust and disrespect with which they were regarded in their past experiences with healthcare and how they flatly refuse to seek any medical attention, however urgently they may require it. The abundance of fear and distrust was palpable. The session concluded that it is important to connect with the community, as sessions like these always do, but how, I wondered, when the community in question was so reluctant to give us the benefit of the doubt.

Similarly, when we as trained medical personnel are posted to rural locations, the locals regard us with doubt and mistrust, often choosing to believe in self proclaimed experts that dole out medications indiscriminately due to greater familiarity. This clearly has the potential to do plenty of damage.

How do we reach across this divide? What is the missing link here? I hope as I progress in my career as a physician, I can find answers to these questions, yet for now I have understood the importance of asking them.

CHAPTER V

The Rollercoaster of my Internship:

-By Dr. Yashaswi Guntupalli (MBBS, Sri Padmavathi Medical College for Women, Tirupati)

Studying medicine was never based on a firm decision of mine. However, it did change my life - for the better! Over time I realised how much I was falling in love with this subject. When I first decided to take up biology in class 10, I remember how unsure I was about it. My belief in my destiny and that it had something beautiful in store steered me to take up the subject anyway.

So, I just followed my heart and there I was! - in a medical college that is 8 hours away from my hometown. It was my first time being away from home. I was a mixed bag of emotions! It was a bittersweet feeling.

My ups and downs during med school had its own set of memories. The reality of being a doctor truly hit me during my INTERNSHIP.

The years passed by so quickly. It was very overwhelming. The thought of working full-time as a student doctor was quite terrifying. I had so many petty questions running in my head. Will patients question me about rare clinical syndromes? Would I be asked to interpret complex scans? What kind of doctor will I become? How will I take death? Etc. I had sweaty palms just thinking about all this.

My internship was a period where I learned so much from my fellow students, my post-graduate seniors, professors, and patients. It was emotionally very turbulent for me, but at the same time, it taught me so many lessons that no textbook ever could.

Experiencing Deaths

The first time I encountered death as an intern, it felt as if the ground had been pulled from under me. Despite all the theoretical knowledge and preparedness, nothing could truly prepare me for the finality of death. It wasn't just the loss of life that hit hard, but the ripple effect it had on the family and friends left behind. I remember standing in the sterile hospital room, the monitors silent, and the weight of the moment pressing down on me. He had been admitted with severe heart failure. Despite all our efforts, despite the advanced technology and knowledge, we couldn't save him. His wife, a kind woman with a warm smile, was inconsolable. Each death left an indelible mark, a mix of sorrow and a renewed resolve to do better for the next patient. I remember the exact moment when I was holding the hand of a grieving spouse, their tears soaking into my scrubs, and realizing the profound impact of our roles as doctors—not just as healers, but as bearers of news that can shatter worlds.

Emotional Lows and Highs

Each day was a roller coaster of emotions. Sleepless nights, endless rounds, and the constant pressure to perform took their toll. There were days when I felt utterly helpless, watching patients deteriorate despite our best efforts. The frustration of not being able to save everyone was a heavy burden. But then there were the highs—those moments when a patient turned a corner, when a child's fever broke, when a long-term patient finally went home, or the successful execution of a complex procedure. These victories, no matter how small, were the light in the often dark tunnel of the internship. These highs acted as beacons that guided me through the darkest times.

Sadness and Empathy

One of the hardest aspects was seeing patients in desperate need and feeling helpless. One particularly grueling night, I was on my 30th hour of no sleep and had an emergency case. An old couple came in with complaints of severe cough and breathlessness to the husband. Our professor suspected PE. I went and told the wife to get a HEPARIN Vial for injecting it into her husband. She opened her little purse and started counting money. Her husband came running from the bed to help her. We told him not to walk but he didn't want to let his wife do everything. I bought the vial with my money. But that night the frustration and helplessness I felt was so intense that I felt the sadness in my bones. The sadness of a mother who couldn't afford her child's treatment, the despair of an elderly man with no family to visit him—these stories were all too common. It was in these moments that I learned the true value of empathy. As much as my medical skills were needed, so too was my ability to listen, to comfort, and to simply be there. Sometimes, the greatest help I could offer was not a prescription, but a reassuring word and a compassionate ear.

The Learning Curve

Every case, every patient, was a learning experience. I quickly realized that medical school had given me the foundation, but the real education came from hands-on experience. There were times I made mistakes, and the guilt was almost unbearable. But with each error came a lesson, and with each lesson, I grew a bit more confident and capable.

Personal Growth

Through the highs and lows, I grew not only as a doctor but as a person. I learned to cope with stress, to manage my emotions, and to find strength in my vulnerabilities. The camaraderie with fellow interns and the guidance of seasoned mentors were invaluable. We shared our triumphs and defeats, finding solace in each other's company. I remember nights in the break room, sharing stories and laughter, those moments of connection were lifelines.

Reflections

Looking back, my internship was a crucible that tested my limits and forged my character. It was a whirlwind of emotions and experiences. It was a period of intense learning, not just about medicine, but about humanity. The experiences shaped my outlook on life and medicine. I faced death, celebrated life, and learned to navigate the complex landscape of emotions that come with being a doctor. Through the highs and lows, I found my calling reaffirmed—despite the overwhelming nature of it all, I knew that this was where I was meant to be. I emerged from it with a deeper understanding of the fragility of life, the importance of empathy, and the relentless pursuit of excellence in the service of others.

Before concluding this chapter of my life, I would like to remark that my internship experience was like a song! - one that I want to play over and over again. Furthermore, there is absolutely nothing about this phase of my life that I would change if I had to go through it all over again.

A favourite saying of mine is "The risk of love is loss, and the price of loss is grief." – Hilary Stanton Zunin.

CHAPTER VI

The Medical School Journey

-By Sai Priya Chandana Mukkamala

Everybody joins medical school with different goals and dreams, but one thing is common: to save lives. Everyone remembers their first day of medical school, well, so do I. I remember being anxious, excited, and having a slight fear, however, now that I think of it, it feels special. The feeling of wearing a white coat for the first time and posing for a picture is a beautiful one. When I entered the dissection hall for the first time, I realized it wasn't easy. The first lectures and the first practical lab classes were all new, but deep down, I knew it was all worth it. It is worth not just to be called a doctor but to be one. As time passed, I enjoyed learning about the normal human body, its functions, its effects on it, diseases, and disorders. After the end of the first year, as I entered the second year, I got to see patients, and interacting with them made me understand the weight of the profession I wanted to pursue. It was not an easy journey; it was pretty hard, but I loved every bit of it. Every chapter and every subject that I learned helped me understand better. Then comes the final year of school. It was the hardest; I can even say that it was one of the toughest times of my life, but I kept pushing myself and got through it all. I can say I fought it right, and I won! I say again, I won, I earned it! DOCTOR!

Then came the time for the internship. The internship was a year of practicing what I learned during my time at school. That one year has made me a better person not only professionally but also personally, mentally, emotionally, and in every other possible way.

I still remember my first day. I was way too anxious because I was going to treat people, and a simple mistake from my side could cost one's life. Even now, I have that fear, but I've gained confidence over time.

There are a few things I will never forget:

~ The first time I administered an IM injection to a patient was memorable, she returned next week for another one, and he specifically wanted me to administer it as it wasn't painful the first time. It made my day.

~ From being picked to dissect a cadaver to assisting in surgery, I realized I had come a long way. The first surgery that I assisted was a right-sided hernioplasty. I still remember the patient's name, and I sutured the surgical site. On POD 2, when the patient came for dressing, my PG appreciated me, saying that the suturing was perfect. It was one of the best compliments I have received to date.

~ A female whose name I still remember was the first patient whom I had admitted to the MICU, she was treated and discharged successfully.

~ Being appreciated for cracking the ECG.

~ It was always a wonderful feeling to see the patients going home after recovering. Later, when they came for a follow-up, they recognized me and asked if I was doing well. They are truly memorable moments.

~ The way patients thank us for treating them is priceless.

And these things gave me a High! Nothing has ever given me the same feeling! And that's what I live for.

>Med school isn't easy, but I did it, and when I can, so can you!

I don't want to stop here. I may or may not become the best doctor in the world; however, I am sure I'll make a good one!

CHAPTER VII

Internship Diaries – Experiencing deaths.

-By Dr.Tulsi Mehta (Intern Doctor, GMERS Medical College, Sola, Ahmedabad)

My life had been quite rosy in medschool. I was unbeknownst to the hardships of the actual world. I only had to worry about my medschool grades, which I managed fairly well.

Until the internship started...

I was super excited for my internship. All the cram work done in the last 4 years was finally going to be put to use.

First day - I enter the medicine ward and I see 20 beds full of patients.

I couldn't wait to examine all the paitents, see their medical records and the treatment provided. The residents taught me hands-on procedures like inserting and removing Foley's catheter, drawing blood from the radial artery for Arterial blood gas analysis(ABGA), inserting the Ryles tube, and using the ECG machine among others.

I found ABGA to be a particularly difficult procedure since I couldn't locate the radial artery easily. Once I tried ABGA in a patient. And I got it in the first try. I was overjoyed. I thanked the patient and the relatives for being cooperative with me. I ran the ABGA sample and it was normal. I assured the patient and her relative that there was nothing to worry about. All night long I kept thinking about how the patient was the first person I was successful in taking ABGA in. She was a teacher to me and she probably didn't even realize it. I will remember her lifelong.

The next morning as I entered the ward, the first thing I got to know was the patient had passed away. I was shocked. A person who was stable till yesterday had passed away due to sudden cardiac arrest.

This was the first time I was experiencing somebody's death — I could not fathom how a person who had been smiling yesterday no longer existed today.

I consoled myself that all those who entered the world had to leave it someday and that I should not be bothered much by it. I continued my work.

2 weeks later I was posted for Casualty duty. A 42-year-old man came with complaints of chest pain late at night. That particular night was a busy one in the casualty area. I was busy taking the vitals of other patients and missed this patient. His wife who accompanied him asked me 2-3 times to check her husband and even held my hand once. I politely told her to wait and as soon as I had attended to a few critical patients, I checked his vitals which were normal. We had his ECG done and checked his Troponin levels. Surprisingly his Troponin levels were normal but ECG was abnormal. The resident diagnosed it as atypical Myocardial infarction(MI) and had the patient admitted.

My casualty duties were going to end that day and I was posted in the ward for night duty from the next day.

My first night duty was uneventful- except for a patient who had some uneasiness due to indigestion and the patient whom I had earlier met in the casualty with atypical MI who had a headache. The wife of the patient who had the MI came to me again and again and held my hand to check her husband. I told her I would come soon as I was busy with another patient. I consulted the resident and gave them appropriate medicines. Around 2 AM I went to the Doctor's room to get some sleep as all patients were stable and the work for the night was done.

I would have barely slept for 15 minutes when I heard the screams of a woman. I looked around the room and saw the patient whose ABGA I had done earlier. She was sitting in her bed. And surprisingly it was the same bed as the ward where she was admitted.

My eyes opened and I stood up. I was experiencing a nightmare. I was seeing and hearing a patient who had died. I drank some water, took deep breaths and tried going back to sleep again.

2nd day of my ward duty, I reached at 8 PM for my night duty. The intern who had the evening duty was nowhere. I thought she must have left. Suddenly she came panting. She told she had gone to the ICCU as a patient had to be transferred. On further inquiring, I found the patient had passed away and it was the same patient with atypical MI.

I was shattered. This was the second death thst I had witnessed in the last 2 weeks. I could only remember the cheerful face of the patient as I was measuring his blood pressure in the casualty. He had asked his wife to calm down and let the doctors do the work.

I could not process his death. I went around the ward and saw the empty bed which was just occupied by him yesterday.

As I was going out of the ward, I noticed the patient's wife. Her eyes were red and swollen from all the crying. I could only imagine how much she would have felt lonely in that moment. I gathered the courage to console her and as I began to ask one of her relatives signalled me to keep quiet. They told she wasn't able to handle her husband's death and repeatedly reminding her would only make matters worse.

I noticed she was still in the same clothes as she was wearing 2 days ago in the casualty.

Somehow my night passed.

I broke down when I reached home. I couldn't keep the thoughts out of my mind. For 3 days, the only thing I could think of was about that patient — his cheerful face, his calmness, the worry on his wife's face, her red swollen eyes after his death.

I was completely dejected for the rest of the week.

Unable to handle it no longer, I asked my senior how she managed to cope with such feelings. She told me," Complete 1 year of your internship and then ask me the same question. "After the ward duty, I was posted in the ICU. The patients there had very few chances of recovering and most of them died. I would feel sad every time a death happened but there was nothing much that I could do.

Over time I accepted that this was going to be a part of my life now. I understood what my senior had been trying to explain to me.

It made me realize how important my job was and how many hopes the patients and their relatives pinned on the doctors. I have heard so many patients tell the intern doctors and resident doctors that they are no less than God to them.

We get so excited seeing a new case of an unusual disease thinking we will get to learn something new today. But in the process, we forget that the patient is a human too just like

you and me. For us, it may be just another sick body, but for the patient, it is a time of experiencing pain both physical and mental. They could be somebody's loved one and one death completely shatters a family.

All the deaths I saw, completely changed my outlook towards how human life is so perishable, you may be healthy but you never know when death may approach.

I have become much more humbled by all my experiences. I hope to be a good human being before being a good doctor and pass on my experiences to my juniors.

CHAPTER VIII

Witnessed a death due to lack of interest from the patient's family members.

-By Kunj Ghantiwala (MBBS, GMC Bhavnagar)

During my internship in the Internal Medicine department at a government hospital, I encountered a harrowing situation that remains deep in my memory to this day. Assigned to the night shift in casualty, I found myself facing a scenario that highlighted the critical role of family support for further management in medical emergencies.

I considered my placement in internal medicine to be a great opportunity as a medical intern eager to obtain practical experience. Even though I had already finished rotations in a number of specialties, such as orthopedics, ophthalmology, obstetrics and gynecology, and ENT, I was most excited about the complexity and variety of situations in internal medicine like taking rounds in the general ward, ICU and doing emergency duty in casualty.

Since there was no emergency medicine department at the hospital, one of my responsibilities in the casualty department was to give symptomatic treatment and order investigations patients who were referred to internal medicine by the medical officer. This required us to be ready as interns to diagnose and start symptomatic treatment for a variety of diseases and we were accompanied by the R1, R2, and R3.

As I write this, the event is still so clear in my mind that I can see it. One evening as my coworkers and I were getting comfortable into our shift, suddenly we heard the sound of an ambulance siren, alerting us to the approach of a serious case. As we hurried to the scene, we discovered a patient who was in trouble. Her symptoms—agitation, confusion, and chest pain—were obviously urgent, even if the medical officer had not made a formal referral. I informed the nurse to prepare the loading dose for MI, give diclo-pentop, and told the EKG guy to do an EKG on the patient. The patient was 73-year-old female. I quickly identified an inferior wall myocardial infarction (MI) using my training, As I found that out I informed the R1 and R1 informed the R2 and R3. Later the diagnosis was confirmed by the R2 and R3. As the R1 just joined the residency and was from a different state, R1 had a language barrier so I was off paper R1. Vitals: pulse - not palpable, BP – not measurable, temperature – extremities were cold by palpation, HR < 58 beats/min, SpO2: 95%, she was only oriented to place. After we made sure that the patient was receiving the appropriate care and meds we ordered she vomited maybe 250 ml of fluid and then she became unconscious. During this rush, I hardly found any relative asking me questions about her prognosis and health, at that time I didn't pay attention to this but normally when a person is having a heart attack patient's relatives would ask so many questions. The patient's relatives were conspicuously absent from the rush of medical activity, though. The patient was scared and alone, even though we tried to find them. Sadly, the patient suffered a heart arrest just as a family member appeared.

We frantically tried to get consent for more intervention from the family, but due to conflicts between the patient's family members, the procedure was so much delayed. They started abusing each other and they were not sure who would give the consent for further management. Despite our greatest attempts and dedication towards the patient, the patient's health worsened and she died as a result of the delay.
Following the experience, I struggled with a flurry of feelings. As I thought about the unnecessary deaths, I was overwhelmed with rage, frustration, and powerlessness. We were helpless against the reckless and irresponsible behavior of family members, even with our more than 100% commitment to save this patient.

This tragic event provided as a painful reminder of how important family support is to patient outcomes. The healthcare workers would give their best to save the patient's life but we also need support from the family.

CHAPTER IX

The Rainy Night at Cardiology

-By Pooja Manjula (MBBS, GMC Vellore)

Working as a Medical Officer in Cardiology right after internship was a bittersweet experience.

All through medical school, I had wanted to experience the rush and adrenaline of saving a patient's life, witnessing the miracle or at least being a part of the team . So when I had the opportunity to work as a cardiology junior doctor in a multi-speciality hospital in my home town, I was exhilarated to say the least.

First few days flew by with me doing my homework meticulously, reading all about ECGs , heart conditions, presenting cases and getting myself involved in audits and QIPs. As time went and I started really working rather than shadowing, I could slowly feel the essence of it. The responsibility and weight that lay like a heavy blanket on my shoulders in this profession smiled at me in all its glory. I kept questioning myself and making up situations in my head about what I would do when that dreaded day would come. That day when I am all alone, with my seniors nowhere in sight, when I would have to take a decision confidently and handle a situation and lead a team. I knew the possibilities would sky rocket when I would start my night duties.

Finally, that day came.

It was apparently a very peaceful morning duty. I joined in for night duty, and opened the ICU door after my daily ritual of a tiny silent prayer. Very few patients. Only 3 beds occupied. I smiled internally. My colleague gave me a very simple handover of the 3 stable patients left in the ICU – all of them were to be shifted to ward in an hour. He bid me goodbye and told me "Lucky you, I bet you can sleep a minimum of 5 hours. Good luck!"

I took a quick rounds of the patients, documented it and sat down for a chit chat with our nursing staff. It was Nurses day. I ordered a small cake for all of us. After all, isn't a night duty in a free ICU worth celebrating? It started to rain heavily outside.

I went back to the doctor's room in hopes of brushing up some topics for my upcoming exam. 30 minutes went by. Right after cutting the call with the Zomato delivery man who informed me he is waiting downstairs, I got that call. The landline number from A & E.

A man in his 30's- Mr.X (name withheld for confidentiality reasons) had presented with some stomach discomfort. ECG is normal. His wife wants cardiology consultation just to be sure. He is absolutely fine and he is asking for aa antacid to go home. I rolled my eyes. "The ER and their ways" I thought to myself. But who was I kidding. I had all the time in the world today, I would go take a look at the ECG, send him home if he's alright, collect my cake and come back – Or so I thought.

I went and examined Mr.X. He was a big man, quite healthy and well built. He smiled at me wide. In his own words, He had always had gastric discomfort that comes and goes. No other risk factors or previous history. No family history. I took a look at his ECG. The first ECG looked fine and I showed the ER consultant just to be on the safe side. He agreed with me. However, while documenting my notes at the nurse's station, I glanced at him. His face seemed to be uncomfortable when no one was around. He wiped his forehead with a towel and quickly smiled at me when he caught me looking. "A repeat ECG and we'll send cardiac enzymes too in some time". I said, I got the cake and kept it back in my room. Something told me I had to be in the ER, even though it was free. I could cut the cake if hopefully all was well and if the enzymes came back negative.

While back at ER, he seemed much more at ease. I explained that we'll have to observe him for safety. He seemed disappointed. He kept going about his lifestyle and diet habits. He was obviously proud and rightfully so. I explained the condition to his family and they all were in for it. As his discomfort had disappeared by now, everyone started talking and sharing more. His family could connect to me and they told me they felt cared for. I was happy. The rain started to pour heavier in all its might. One of the reasons for a relatively calm night. The second ECG was taken. It looked normal at first sight. Then I quickly compared it with the last one, and I noticed it. Like a sneaky devil, the tiniest J point elevation in leads 11, 111, avF. It was so tiny, I had to see again and again to make sure my eyes weren't playing tricks on me. I felt a pit in my tummy. I immediately showed it to the ER consultant who was as shocked as me. Loading dose of antiplatelets were given immediately, he still had no pain. My cardiology consultant was informed immediately. While explaining the procedures and what it might be to him, he stared at me. Serial ECGs confirmed that it was indeed, an inferior wall MI.

While shifting him to the catheter lab, He still looked quite puzzled. "Will I be fine?" A question that all doctors dread. "Be brave. You have got this" I said as they wheeled him in. Of course he will be. His family was shattered, in disbelief. But thousands of cases have gone into these same 4 walled catheter lab and come out just fine. He will too. I told myself. Till I heard the alarm.

I remember running in with the PPE, to see someone hovering over him, offering CPR. The monitor showed broad regular complexes. VT. Sounds of shock and hustle and shouts. I took over and gave CPR all the while feeling numb inside. I couldn't look at him. It felt personal. He was connected to the ventilator and I brainstormed how I would tell his family when I heard someone shout "Theres a PULSE!" I could hear and feel the relief in that catheter lab. The sweaty doctors, Exhausted nurses, physicians and the one thing that bound all of us together. That little invisible smile of relief and gratitude.

He was quickly wheeled back to the ICU where he was on ventilator, sedated for a number of days. He was the first one I would check on first thing when I came for my duties. Urine output that kept improving, ECGs and BP that kept getting better, Response that started slowly... and one day, as I prayed and entered the ICU again, I saw him lie there peacefully with no tubes attached, staring at the ceiling, as he slowly turned to look at me... and smiled. At that moment I felt I had endured all I did these 6 years for this one day.

That one day taught me about the unpredictability of life. Seeing life slip away from you so fast, seeing the fear of death first hand. Seeing grief, seeing prayers, seeing love, seeing gratitude. None of the cases I had seen in internship, none of the many deaths I had declared, had stirred up such an emotion in me. Maybe the fact that it was someone completely healthy, like me, like my loved ones. Maybe the conversations. I could only assume. But if there's something my few months in Cardiology has taught me, its only this.

Live every moment like it's your last. Celebrate tiny victories. Do things that make your soul smile. Because tomorrow, may never come.

CHAPTER X

Breathing in Danger: The Invisible Threat to Our Children's Health

-By Dr. Jahanvi Grover (MBBS, PGIMS Rohtak)

Growing up in Delhi, I've never seen a bluer sky than in my dreams. The haze of pollution has been an unwelcome companion, etching a grim reality into my consciousness. As a medical student, I've delved deep into the data and stories behind this pervasive issue, and the picture is both alarming and heartbreaking.

Air pollution, an insidious force, wreaks havoc on the health of our youngest and most vulnerable. Recent statistics from 2024 paint a dire picture: over 90% of children worldwide breathe in toxic air daily, with devastating consequences. In Delhi alone, the particulate matter (PM2.5) levels often exceed safe limits by several times, a reality that translates into an array of health issues for children, from asthma to impaired cognitive development.

Anecdotal experiences underscore these statistics. I recall my little cousin, barely five, struggling with severe asthma attacks every winter. Each episode was a grim reminder of the air quality crisis that looms over our city. My Grandfather, who has chronic asthma, faces a particularly tough time during the months of Diwali when fireworks further deteriorate the air quality.

In response to this, we installed an air filter at home. This device has been a lifeline, especially for my Grandfather. It significantly reduces indoor air pollutants, providing him with much-needed relief during peak pollution periods. Since using the air filter, his asthma attacks have lessened, and he can breathe more easily even during the worst smog days. However, while air filters improve indoor air quality, they also present a conflicting benefit by creating a false sense of security. The root of the problem—outdoor air pollution—remains unaddressed, highlighting the need for broader environmental solutions.

The World Health Organization (WHO) has recognized the urgency of this crisis. In their latest initiatives, they have introduced stricter air quality guidelines and launched programs aimed at reducing emissions and promoting cleaner technologies. These measures are a beacon of hope, but the road ahead remains long and arduous.

In India, the government has rolled out several new schemes to combat air pollution and raise awareness. The National Clean Air Programme (NCAP) has set a target to reduce PM2.5 levels by 20-30% by 2024. Additionally, the 'Green India Mission' focuses on increasing green cover to absorb pollutants, while the 'Pradhan Mantri Ujjwala Yojana' promotes the use of clean cooking fuel to reduce indoor air pollution. These initiatives, combined with public awareness campaigns, aim to create a sustainable and healthier environment for future generations.

Recent studies corroborate the severe impacts of air pollution on children's health. A 2024 study published in The Lancet highlights a direct correlation between high levels of air pollution and increased cases of respiratory and cardiovascular diseases in children. Another study from the Journal of Paediatrics links air pollution exposure to significant delays in neurodevelopmental milestones.

As a Delhite and an aspiring doctor, I am deeply moved by these findings. The bluer skies I dream of aren't just about aesthetic beauty; they represent a future where children can breathe freely, grow healthily, and live fully. Our collective efforts, guided by rigorous science and compassionate policies, can turn this dream into reality.

CHAPTER XI

Understanding Cervical Most Cancers and The Impact of HPV Vaccination

-By Dr. Yash Bahuguna (MS, DNB OBGY, MUHS)

Cervical cancer is an important health concern internationally, affecting women of various ages and backgrounds. But the best part is that we have a way to prevent it: the Human Papillomavirus (HPV) vaccine. Let's dive into how cervical cancers and the HPV vaccine are related and understand how the vaccine can help reduce the prevalence of this disease.

The link among HPV and cervical most cancers:

HPV is a group of viruses, there are virtually over 2 hundred and a number of them are related to maximum cervical cancers. It is commonly spread via sexual contact. Most of the time, your immune system can clear HPV without any problems, but in case you get a non-stop contamination with excessive-threat sorts of HPV, it is able to cause changes in your cervical cells that would later develop into cervical cancer.

Global effect of cervical cancer:

According to the World Health Organization (WHO), cervical cancer is the fourth maximum not unusual most cancers amongst ladies in the arena. In 2020 alone, there have been approximately 604,000 new cases and 342,000 deaths. The burden of cervical cancer is in particular extreme in low- and middle-income countries, together with India, where entry to screening and remedy might not be as easy as in high-income locations which includes the US and the UK.

How the HPV vaccination enables:

Vaccination against HPV is a important step to forestall cervical most cancers. It mainly goals the most uncommon excessive-risk types of HPV which can be related to most cervical cancers, Types 16, 18. By getting the vaccine, your immune system will make antibodies towards these precise kinds of HPV, allowing it to combat the infection and prevent most cervical cancers from developing later .

How effective are HPV vaccines?

Research has shown that HPV vaccines are powerful in decreasing the hazard of getting HPV and related illnesses, such as maximum cervical cancers.

- The bivalent HPV vaccine, which protects from HPV types 16 and 18, has been confirmed to be about 80% effective in preventing chronic HPV infection and the unsightly precancerous lesions. [1]

- The quadrivalent HPV vaccine, which targets HPV variants 6, 11, 16 and 18, has been shown to be about 90% effective in stopping infections with particular HPV subtypes and related diseases, inclusive of cervical precancer and genital warts. [2]

Impact of vaccination applications:

Countries implementing comprehensive HPV vaccination packages have seen several most important upgrades in the rates of HPV contamination and related cervical troubles. Check out those:

- Australia commenced its countrywide HPV vaccination in 2007 and for the reason that then they have obtained a proposal for an wonderful 77% drop in HPV among younger girls aged 18-24. [3]

- HPV vaccination has also made a huge difference in America. A have a look at published in JAMA found that among women aged 14-19, the superiority of the vaccine form of HPV decreased via 88% from 2006 to 2017, all because of the intiation of the HPV vaccine. [4]

HPV vaccination is a game-changer in relation to preventing most cervical cancers. It is strong and makes a real effect within the fight against this cancer.

Vaccine coverage:

Although HPV vaccination has been introduced with many blessings, global coverage remains choppy. Factors which include price, health infrastructure, getting access and public recognition have an impact on access to HPV vaccination. It could be very vital to make efforts to increase vaccine coverage, in particular in underserved areas along with rural agencies, to maximize the effect of HPV vaccination in stopping most cervical cancers.

Conclusion:

In summary, HPV vaccination is an vital approach to decreasing the load of maximum cervical cancers internationally. By stopping HPV contamination and subsequent cervical abnormalities, vaccination programs play a main role in lowering the prevalence and mortality of most kinds of cervical cancer. It is essential to stick and push for better coverage and vaccine availability to acquire large reductions in cervical cancer instances and improve women's health internationally.

Reference:

[1] World Health Organization. (n.D.). Human papillomavirus (HPV) and cervical cancer. Retrieved from https://www.Who.Int/immunization/illnesses/hpv/en/

[2] Centers for Disease Control and Prevention. (2021). HPV vaccine statistics for medical doctors - Fact sheet. Retrieved from https://www.Cdc.Gov/vaccines/vpd/hpv/hcp/efficacy.Html

[3] Centers for Disease Control and Prevention. (n.D.). Six motives to get your child the HPV vaccine. Retrieved from https://www.Cdc.Gov/hpv/mother and father/vaccine/six-motives.Html

[4] Markowitz, L.E., et al. (2018). Declines in human papillomavirus (HPV) occurrence amongst young women following creation of the HPV

vaccine in the United States, National Health and Nutrition Examination Surveys, 2003-2014. JAMA, 319(7), 748-750. Retrieved from https://www.Cdc.Gov/mmwr/volumes/sixty seven/wr/mm6724a4.Html

Surgical Approaches to Regenerative Wound Healing: A Comparative Review of Autologous Fat Grafting versus Flap Surgery

-By Rachel (3rd year medical student, USMF, Moldova)

Introduction

Skin is the biggest organ in the human body that protects and serves as a barrier to the external world. Burns, persistent wounds, and skin injections are all difficult to treat and control, and they are costly for healthcare systems around the world. Extended burns have restricted donor-site skin availability and cause high donor-site morbidity. Obesity and diabetes are associated with an increase in the occurrence of chronic wounds. These are non-healing wounds that can impede the skin's physiological function, resulting in morbidity and even death. Despite the findings, the care of chronic wounds remains unsatisfactory, and there is a need for treatment approaches that may be implemented early with complete wound coverage while preserving normal skin function. (1,2)

Autologous Fat Grafting

An innovative method of treating deep wounds is described by Rangaswamy M. in a study titled "A New Concept and Potential Alternative to Flaps." It involves a simple regenerative technique that forms a triple-layer matrix consisting of collagen dressing, autologous fat, and platelet-rich fibrin matrix (PRFM) to bridge wounds and encourage quick in situ regeneration of vascularized tissue cover, even over the bone. This method has shown success in three case studies. (3)

In order to replace autologous split-thickness skin grafts for tissue regeneration, 3D bioprinting was developed. The method mimics the extracellular matrix by carefully choosing bioinks (6).

Flap Surgery

The ultimate objective of tissue regeneration and flap surgery is to cover and fill the skin while vascularizing the bone. Small amounts of bone can be restored by tissue regeneration, but there are a number of disadvantages, such as cost and availability. (3)

Innovations such as acellular fish skin grafts with collagen, fibrin, and proteoglycans offer the advantage of reducing discomfort, dressing changes, and wound healing while also being more economical. According to studies, AFS can be employed in a variety of clinical settings, including neovaginoplasty in patients with Mayer-Rokitansky-Küster-Hauser syndrome, calciphylaxis, necrotic angiodermatitis, and chronic diabetic foot ulcers. (2)

In regenerative medicine, the use of stem cells and micrografting are crucial. When managing significant burns, the regenerate micrografting technique proves to be efficacious in burn therapy. (4)

Silk has many uses in medicine because of its strength, biocompatibility, and adaptability. It can be applied to bone treatments when mixed with hydrogels. When mixed in certain ways, it also possesses bioactive qualities, including antibacterial and anti-inflammatory effects. (5)

Conclusion:

Although traditional methods like autologous fat grating and flap surgery remain important, there have been numerous innovative advancements in wound management with improved outcomes and a reduction in burden.

References –

1. Kim HS, Sun X, Lee JH, Kim HW, Fu X, Leong KW. Advanced drug delivery systems and artificial skin grafts for skin wound healing. Adv Drug Deliv Rev. 2019 Jun;146:209-239. doi: 10.1016/j.addr.2018.12.014. Epub 2018 Dec 31. PMID: 30605737.
2. Luze H, Nischwitz SP, Smolle C, Zrim R, Kamolz LP. The Use of Acellular Fish Skin Grafts in Burn Wound Management-A Systematic Review. Medicina (Kaunas). 2022 Jul 9;58(7):912. doi: 10.3390/medicina58070912. PMID: 35888631; PMCID: PMC9323726.
3. Rangaswamy M. Regenerative Wound Healing by Open Grafting of Autologous Fat and PRP-Gel - A New Concept and Potential Alternative to Flaps. Plast Reconstr Surg Glob Open. 2021 Jan 25;9(1):e3349. doi: 10.1097/GOX.0000000000003349. PMID: 33564580; PMCID: PMC7859317.
4. Astarita C, Arora CL, Trovato L. Tissue regeneration: an overview from stem cells to micrografts. J Int Med Res. 2020 Jun;48(6):300060520914794. doi: .10.1177/0300060520914794. PMID: 32536230; PMCID: PMC7297485.
5. Koczoń P, Dąbrowska A, Laskowska E, Łabuz M, Maj K, Masztakowski J, Bartyzel BJ, Bryś A, Bryś J, Gruczyńska-Sękowska E. Applications of Silk Fibroin in Human and Veterinary
6. Masri S, Zawani M, Zulkiflee I, Salleh A, Fadilah NIM, Maarof M, Wen APY, Duman F, Tabata Y, Aziz IA, Bt Hj Idrus R, Fauzi MB. Cellular Interaction of Human Skin Cells towards Natural Bioink via 3D-Bioprinting Technologies for Chronic Wound: A Comprehensive Review. Int J Mol Sci. 2022 Jan 1;23(1):476. doi: 10.3390/ijms23010476. PMID: 35008902; PMCID: PMC8745539.

CHAPTER XIII

Cancer Prevention and Control in India

Here we outline some of the most critical actions to help realize the global objectives:
-By Mridul Pandey (3rd year medical student, Sri Guru Ram Rai Institute of Medical and Health Sciences)

Introduction

Cancer is one of the biggest health issues of the world; in India, oneness has to be accorded to Non-Communicable diseases issues; hence Cancer. Therefore, active development and implementation of important strategies for cancer prevention and control are needed to meet the goals of the SDG by the year 2030.

1. Reviewing National Efforts

India depends on measures or programs such as the National Cancer Control Program (NCCP) against cancer. Summing up, one can state that certain advancements have been observed; however, certain issues require further work. These programs should be audited to address the following: determine areas of inefficiency and vulnerability, enhance infrastructure, diagnose delays, and enhance the provision of treatment.

2. Strengthening Primary Health Care

Primary Health Care (PHC) serve as the backbone for any health care system. Well-established systems of PHC mean early identification of cancer, which predicts better treatment results and low mortality rates among patients. Education of health care professionals must be conducted, initiation of cancer preventive screenings must be made, and governmental organizations and other responsible bodies must include cancer care in primary health care services. Telemedicine can reach people that otherwise cannot be reached easily.

3. Engaging Communities

Cultural beliefs affect people's choice for treatment. In order to get the public involved in cancer prevention, it is necessary to facilitate contacts with communities. Utilizing culturally appropriate promotional strategies, CHWs, and local opinion influencers can help to promote people's compliance with the screenings. Eradicating stigma that is associate with such diseases such as cancer also has to be done.

4. Synthesis of Ayurveda Systems of Medicine and the Modern Medicine

There is much knowledge which is present in the Ayurvedic tradition of India that could help to enrich people's lives alongside from the approaches used in modern medicine. Conducting a study on how Ayurvedic system of medicine can be complementary to the conventional method of treatment may prove fruitful. More effort should be directed to evaluate findings on the use of herbs and other Non-Pharmacologic Interventions and Cancer Prevention.

5. Encouraging Ongoing Research

Its importance is rooted in the fact that cancer trends are dynamic, hence regular research and updates are called for. Reading epidemiology, genetics, or information from clinical trials, which referred to and used in many disciplines, is significant. It shows that synergy between medical workers and academics as well as governments means that the best interventions will be developed.

Conclusion

In view of the achievement of the Third SDG of health and wellbeing, cancer prevention and control must be enhanced. Research supports the notion that increased spending in the community, engagement, and collaborations will go a long way in eradicating this disease.

References:

1. Ramani VK, Jayanna K, Naik R. A commentary on cancer prevention and control in India: Priorities for realizing SDGs. Health Sci Rep. 2023 Feb;6(2):e1126. doi: 10.1002/hsr2.1126. (https://europepmc.org/article/MED/36824617)

CHAPTER XIV

Field Cancerization: Unveiling the Devastating Impact of Tobacco: A Mini-Review

- Dr. Krutika Mahendra Gohil (MBBS, HBTMC and Dr. R.N. Cooper Municipal General Hospital, Mumbai)

Dr. Jyothika Venkataswamy Reddy (MBBS, Chamarajanagar Institute of Medical Sciences)

Introduction:

One intriguing and multifaceted concept in oncology is "field cancerization," which refers to the pervasiveness of precancerous cellular alterations in a certain tissue or organ that pave the way for several primary malignancies. The notion of field cancerization is supported by the emergence of recurrences and secondary primary tumors, even in cases where surgical margins are histopathologically tumor-free. Slaughter et al introduced the term 'field cancerization' in oral cancers in 1953 [1]. Chronic exposure to carcinogens like tobacco smoke in the aerodigestive tract can elicit a cascade of mutations and epigenetic modifications that can lead to field cancerization. Field cancerization is a well-known mechanism that turns an existing precancerous lesion into cancer. This is called a field effect (field defect). In patients with head and neck cancer, tobacco use raises the probability of concurrent or subsequent disease.

Oral Field Cancerization:

Field cancerization encompasses the emergence of cancer in multiple areas of precancerous modifications, the presence of abnormal tissue surrounding the primary tumor, and oral cancer frequently consisting of numerous independent lesions that may merge. Additionally, the persistence of abnormal tissue even after surgery can account for the possibility of second primary tumors (SPT) [2].

A set of diagnostic criteria for multiple primary carcinomas was first developed by Warren and Gates [3] and then revised by Hong et al. [4].

a) Each neoplasm must be distinct and anatomically separate.

b) A probability of a second primary carcinoma representing a metastasis or a local relapse should be excluded.

The epithelium in the aerodigestive tract undergoes priming due to prolonged exposure to carcinogens, leading to the development of multifocal carcinomas stemming from distinct mutations occurring independently within the preconditioned epithelium.

Model of Field Cancerization:

A stem cell that undergoes one or more genetic and epigenetic changes is the first step in the carcinogenesis process. A clone of genetically modified cells then develops into a patch or a cluster. [5]

The carcinogenesis model has a monoclonal origin and consists of three essential steps:[6]

Phase one (patch formation): a single stem cell (patch) is transformed into a clone, a collection of cells bearing genetic changes but without an appropriate growth control pattern.

Phase two (clonal expansion): more genetic changes arise, the patch multiplies by utilizing its increased growth capability, and it forms a field that pushes aside the healthy epithelium.

Phase three (transition to tumor): the field or clone finally develops into an overt carcinoma with metastases and invasive development.

Mechanism:

Tobacco smoke contains polycyclic aromatic hydrocarbons (PAHs) and nitrosamines, which can provoke genetic mutations and epigenetic changes in cells lining the aerodigestive tract. DNA damage consequently causes mutations in key oncogenes and tumor suppressor genes, such as TP53, KRAS, and PIK3CA. Tobacco use can prompt DNA methylation and histone modifications, inducing altered gene expression and thus initiating the cascade of carcinogenesis. Mutated cells undergo clonal proliferation, giving rise to an extensive population of mutated cells with a higher propensity for malignant transformation. Chronic inflammation and changes triggered by tobacco exposure foster a pro-carcinogenic environment, facilitating cancer development in the affected field.

Two hypotheses have been proposed to describe the emergence of carcinomas in particular locations. According to one theory, multiple squamous cell lesions arise autonomously as a consequence of simultaneous exposure of the oral cavity to carcinogens, resulting in diverse genetic abnormalities across the entire region [1]. An alternative hypothesis suggests that the genesis of multiple lesions stems from the migration of dysplastic and modified cells [7].

Clinical Importance and Management:

Based on the identification of molecular fingerprints in a genetically altered but histologically normal field known as the peri-tumoral cancer field, this cancer-prone field can be identified. Tumor markers specific to a particular tumor are needed for this. Finding these trustworthy tumor biomarkers will therefore aid in tracking the tumor's development and stop pre-malignant lesions from developing into aggressive cancer. [8]
Loss of heterozygosity, microsatellite changes, chromosomal instability, and p53 gene mutations are among the frequently used markers. These are typically found by polymerase chain reaction, immunohistochemistry,

and in situ hybridization.[9]

The management approach is predicated on the idea that the morphologically changed area will be the site of oral malignancies [10]. Nevertheless, recent data indicates that the mucosa next to it, which appears clinically normal, also carries genetic abnormalities related to early malignant transformation. [11]

Advice and encouragement on quitting habits during follow-up appointments is fundamental. Further genetic alterations in the precancer areas will result from continuous exposure to tobacco toxins. Long-term patient monitoring and follow-up should be prioritized. Also, examining the entire oral cavity, not just the lesional area, should be prioritized.

Conclusion:

Field cancerization predisposes large expanses of tissue to malignant transformation, thus entailing a radical shift in cancer diagnosis, prevention, and management strategies. Field cancerization is directly linked to tobacco consumption, alcohol, smoking, flushing reactions, and high-temperature food consumption. Giving up alcohol and tobacco greatly lowers the chance of developing a second primary cancer. By embracing a holistic view, clinicians can effectively mitigate the risk of cancer and improve patient prognosis. The study of field cancerization expands our understanding of carcinogenesis and complements it to combat this multifaceted disease.

References:

1. Slaughter DP, Southwick HW, Smejkal W. Field cancerization in oral stratified squamous epithelium; clinical implications of multicentric origin Cancer. 1953;6:963–8

2. Braakhuis BJ, Tabor M, Kummer JA, Leemans CR, Brakenhoff R. A genetic explanation of Slaughter's concept of field cancerization: Evidence and clinical implications Cancer Res. 2003;63:1727–30

3. Warren S, Gates O (1932) Multiple primary malignant tumours: A survey of the literature and a statistical study. Am J Cancer 16: 1358-1414.

4. Hong WK, Lippman SM, Itri LM, Karp DD, Lee JS, et al. (1990) Prevention of second primary tumors with isotretinoin in squamous-cell carcinoma of the head and neck. N Engl J Med 323(12): 795-801.

5. Tabor MP, Brakenhoff RH, van Houten VM, Kummer JA, Snel MH, Snijders PJ, Snow GB, Leemans CR, Braakhuis BJ. Persistence of genetically altered fields in head and neck cancer patients: biological and clinical implications. Clin Cancer Res. 2001 Jun;7(6):1523-32. PMID: 11410486.

6. Izzo JG, Papadimitrakopoulou VA, Li XQ, Ibarguen H, Lee JS, Ro JY, El-Naggar A, Hong WK, Hittelman WN. Dysregulated cyclin D1 expression early in head and neck tumorigenesis: in vivo evidence for an association with subsequent gene amplification. Oncogene. 1998 Nov 5;17(18):2313-22. doi: 10.1038/sj.onc.1202153. PMID: 9811462.

7. Corio R, Lee D, Greenberg B, Koch W, Sidransky D, et al. (1996) Genetic Progression model for head and neck cancer: implication for field cancerization. Cancer Res 56(11): 2488-2492.

8. Hong WK, Endicott J, Itri LM, Doos W, Batsakis JG, Bell R, Fofonoff S, Byers R, Atkinson EN, Vaughan C, et al. 13-cis-retinoic acid in the treatment of oral leukoplakia. N Engl J Med. 1986 Dec 11;315(24):1501-5. doi: 10.1056/NEJM198612113152401. PMID: 3537787.

9. Angadi PV, Savitha JK, Rao SS, Sivaranjini Y. Oral field cancerization: current evidence and future perspectives. Oral Maxillofac Surg. 2012 Jun;16(2):171-80. doi: 10.1007/s10006-012-0317-x. Epub 2012 Feb 22. PMID: 22354325.

10. Neville B, Douglas D, Carl D, Allen Angela CI, editors. Oral and Maxillofacial Pathology. 1st ed. South Asia: Elsevier India; 2015. [Google Scholar]

11. Lydiatt WM, Anderson PE, Bazzana T, Casale M, Hughes CJ, Huvos AG, Lydiatt DD, Schantz SP. Molecular support for field cancerization in the head and neck. Cancer. 1998 Apr 1;82(7):1376-80. PMID: 9529031.

CHAPTER XV

The Rise of Menstrual Disorders in the Modern Era: An In-Depth Look

-By Dr. Yash Bahuguna (MS, DNB OBGY)

Introduction:

So, here's the deal: menstrual disorders have become a major concern for women's health worldwide in recent times. These disorders cover a range of conditions like irregular periods, polycystic ovary syndrome (PCOS), premenstrual syndrome (PMS), and painful periods (dysmenorrhea). Figuring out what's causing the rise in these disorders is crucial for effective prevention and management. In this analysis, we're diving deep into the influences of lifestyle, environmental toxins, stress, and societal attitudes on menstrual health. We'll be drawing on the latest research and expert insights to give you the lowdown.

Lifestyle Factors:

Let's talk about how our modern diet is playing a big role in the development of menstrual disorders. Eating a lot of processed foods, sugary snacks, and unhealthy fats messes with our hormones and throws off our menstrual cycles. For example, a study by Gaskins et al. (2019) found that young women who drank a lot of sugary drinks were more likely to have irregular periods.

Also, our sedentary lifestyle these days is a real bummer for our hormones and periods. Not getting enough exercise leads to more body fat and insulin resistance, both of which can mess up our menstrual function (Rich-Edwards et al., 2002). Getting regular exercise in our daily routine can help keep our hormones in check and ease menstrual symptoms.

Environmental Toxins:

Now, let's talk about the not-so-friendly chemicals lurking in our modern environment. These endocrine-disrupting chemicals (EDCs) found in plastics, pesticides, and personal care products are a real threat to our reproductive health. They mess with our hormones and contribute to menstrual disorders (Gore et al., 2015). One common culprit is bisphenol A (BPA), which is found in a lot of plastics and has been linked to messed-up periods and reduced fertility (Rochester, 2013).

What's even scarier is that exposure to these environmental toxins during critical periods of development, like when we're in our mom's womb or during early childhood, can have long-lasting effects on our reproductive health. A study by Casas et al. (2016) found that prenatal exposure to certain chemicals called phthalates was linked to messed-up periods and earlier age at first period in girls.

Stress and Psychosocial Factors:

Okay, let's talk about stress and how it messes with our menstrual health. The pressures of modern life, like work stress, money worries, and social expectations, really take a toll on our periods. Chronic stress messes with a system in our body called the hypothalamic-pituitary-adrenal (HPA) axis, which controls our menstrual cycle (Wissner-Gross & Bonsall, 2006). Research shows that women in high-stress jobs are more likely to have irregular periods compared to those in less stressful jobs (Reid et al., 2014).

On top of that, the way society looks at periods can make things even worse. Menstrual stigma, which is still a thing in many cultures, makes us feel ashamed and secretive about our periods. This adds to the stress and anxiety we feel about our menstrual cycles (Chrisler et al., 2013). We need to tackle this stigma head-on through education and advocacy efforts to promote positive menstrual health.

Sociocultural Factors:

Hey there! When it comes to menstrual disorders, there are some sociocultural influences that play a role. Factors like socioeconomic status, access to healthcare, and cultural norms can all have an impact. Unfortunately, women from marginalized communities may face additional barriers to getting the menstrual health resources they need. This can lead to untreated symptoms and complications (Van Eijk et al., 2016). On top of that, cultural beliefs and practices around menstruation can affect how women view their own menstrual health and influence their actions when seeking help.

But here's the thing: disparities in menstrual health education can lead to a lot of misinformation and misunderstandings about periods. And that, in turn, can cause delays in diagnosing and treating menstrual disorders. That's why it's super important to integrate comprehensive menstrual health education into school curricula and healthcare settings. When women have all the facts, they can make informed decisions about their reproductive health.

To wrap things up, the rise of menstrual disorders in our modern era is a complex issue. There are a bunch of factors at play, like lifestyle choices, exposure to environmental toxins, stress, and sociocultural attitudes. To tackle this, we need a multi-pronged approach. We're talking public health interventions, policy changes, and community-based initiatives. By promoting healthy habits, reducing exposure to toxins, and addressing the stressors in our lives, we can make a real difference in the burden that menstrual disorders place on women's health and well-being.

References:

- Casas, M., Valvi, D., Ballesteros-Gomez, A., Gascon, M., Fernández, M. F., Garcia-Esteban, R., ... & Vrijheid, M. (2016). Exposure to bisphenol A and phthalates during pregnancy and offspring size at birth. Environmental Research, 150, 119-125.

- Chrisler, J. C., Gorman, J. A., & Manion, J. (2013). Measuring menstrual cycle experiences: Development of the menstrual symptom questionnaire. Health Care for Women International, 34(10), 841–860.

- Gaskins, A. J., Williams, P. L., Keller, M. G., Souter, I., Hauser, R., & Chavarro, J. E. (2019). Association between sugar-sweetened beverage intake and age at menarche: The project Viva cohort. Pediatric Obesity,

14(1), e12460.

- Gore, A. C., Chappell, V. A., Fenton, S. E., Flaws, J. A., Nadal, A., Prins, G. S., ... Zoeller, R. T. (2015). EDC-2: The Endocrine Society's Second Scientific Statement on Endocrine-Disrupting Chemicals. Endocrine Reviews, 36(6), E1–E150.

- Reid, K. M., Taylor, M. G., & Thompson, J. M. (2014). The stressors of working-class mothers of infants: A qualitative exploration of their accounts. Journal of Reproductive and Infant Psychology, 32(3), 285–299.

- Rochester, J. R. (2013). Bisphenol A and human health: A review of the literature. Reproductive Toxicology, 42, 132–155.

- Van Eijk, A. M., Sivakami, M., Thakkar, M. B., Bauman, A., & Laserson, K. F. (2016). Menstrual hygiene management among adolescent girls in India: A systematic review and meta-analysis. BMJ Open, 6(3), e010290.

CHAPTER XVI

TZIELD (TEPLIZUMAB) Altering The Course of Diabetes Type 1

-By Jeshtha Chaudhari (Final year MBBS student KIMS Karad)

Introduction:

Type 1 diabetes mellitus (T1DM) is an autoimmune disorder leading to the selective destruction of pancreatic beta-cells, ultimately leading to loss of insulin production. Individuals with T1DM require lifelong insulin replacement therapy through use of multiple daily insulin injections or insulin pumps. Without insulin, diabetic ketoacidosis may develop and is fatal if left untreated.

T1DM is predominately diagnosed in children and adolescents below or equal to 18 years of age, although it can have its onset at any age. Although the exact aetiology of T1D is still unknown, researchers believe there is a genetic predisposition with a strong link with specific HLA (DR and DQ) alleles.

Stages of diabetes type 1:

The development of T1D occurs in 3 stages.

Stage 1 is asymptomatic and characterised by normal fasting glucose, normal glucose tolerance, and the presence of ≥2 pancreatic autoantibodies.

Stage 2 diagnostic criteria include the presence of pancreatic autoantibodies (usually multiple) and dysglycemia: impaired fasting glucose (fasting glucose 100 to 125 mg/dL) or impaired glucose tolerance (2-hour post-75 gm glucose load glucose 140 to 199 mg/dL) or an HbA1c

5.7% to 6.4%. Individuals remain asymptomatic.

In stage 3, there is diabetes, defined by hyperglycemia (random glucose ≥200 mg/dL) with clinical symptoms, fasting glucose ≥126 mg/dL, glucose ≥200 mg/dL two hours after ingesting 75 g of glucose during an oral glucose tolerance test and/or HbA1c ≥6.5%. If the individual lacks classic symptoms of hyperglycemia or hyperglycemic crisis, it is recommended that two tests be performed (simultaneously or at different times) to confirm the diagnosis.

Hence to delay the prognosis of the stage 2 to stage 3 a drug named TEPLIZUMAB is introduced by preserving beta cell function .

The goal of teplizumab is to delay the onset of clinical diabetes, with the classic symptoms of excessive urination and thirst and other complications, as long as possible. Researchers say the drug postpones the median onset of the disease by at least two years.

Recent Findings:

In November 2022, teplizumab-mzwv (TZIELD; Provention Bio, Inc., a Sanofi Company, Red Bank, NJ) became the first drug approved to change the progression of autoimmunity in type 1 diabetes (i.e., to delay the onset of stage 3 type 1 diabetes in adults and children age ≥8 years with stage 2 disease). The approval of teplizumab represents the first drug approval for the delay of any autoimmune disease in patients before clinical onset. Decades of studies preceded the approval of teplizumab, beginning with preclinical studies followed by six clinical trials, including five in patients after clinical diagnosis (stage 3) and one in patients before clinical diagnosis (stage 2) who had two or more pancreatic islet autoantibodies and dysglycemia.

Teplizumab is a humanized immunoglobulin G1 monoclonal antibody that binds with high affinity to the ε chain of CD3. Its complementarity-determining region is derived from ortho kung T3 (OKT3), the first monoclonal antibody licensed for human use for acute solid graft rejection. OKT3 was humanized to minimize immunogenicity. Two Leu→Ala substitutions in the Fc region were introduced to minimize Fc-receptor binding, resulting in 100- to 1,000-fold reduction in T-cell activation, T-cell proliferation, and cytokine release in human peripheral blood mononuclear cell cultures compared with OKT3 . Early studies of its mechanism showed that partial agonism led to effects on CD8+ T cells integral to autoimmune-mediated destruction of pancreatic β-cells .

The approved label for TZIELD includes warnings and precautions for serious infections, lymphopenia, hypersensitivity reactions, and vaccinations. The safety profile of teplizumab was characterised by mild to moderate AEs that were self-limited. Higher rates of serious infections were observed, although overall rates of infections were similar between treatment groups. A majority of teplizumab-treated patients developed lymphopenia , which resolved even while dosing continued and without treatment interruption . Importantly, the development of transient lymphopenia did not seem to be associated with an overall increased risk of infection. Although not included in the integrated analysis, 7-year follow-up of patients in the AbATE study showed no increased risk of infections and no malignancies

There are several important features that distinguish teplizumab from other therapies previously tested in patients with type 1 diabetes.

First, teplizumab was administered in two defined intravenous courses (12 days each), and a more rapid recovery of circulating immune cells occurred after treatment than has been shown to occur with therapies given continuously or with those that result in prolonged cell depletion. The long-term effects of teplizumab do not appear to entail chronic immunosuppression. The clinical evidence for recovery of immune function was apparent in this trial from the resolution of EBV reactivation and Covid-19 in patients treated with teplizumab.

Second, the effects of teplizumab appeared to be prolonged. Teplizumab is thought to induce partial CD8+ T-cell exhaustion that impedes T-cell function.Such a mechanism may affect certain T cells, which have relatively weak engagement with their targets, such as autoreactive cells, and thus, we speculate, may be more easily modulated. These features appeared to be consistent with functional immune tolerance (i.e., the restoration of unresponsiveness to one's own tissues [or self-antigens] while maintaining defensive immune responses).

Previous preclinical studies and analyses of cells from teplizumab-treated patients have suggested that this partial agonist signal, which leads to changes in the composition of differentiation and activation within circulating T cells may lead to partial exhaustion of CD8+ T cells, which has been associated with reduced cytokine production after activation. Indeed, investigations of patients from the AbATE and TN-10 studies showed that the CD8+TIGIT+KLRG1+ memory T cells from teplizumab-treated patients showed signs of exhaustion and produced lower levels of the inflammatory cytokines tumour necrosis factor-α and interferon-γ, which are associated with T cell–mediated β-cell death . Because teplizumab targets activated effector cells and spares regulatory T cells and memory T cells against previously encountered pathogens, the preservation of β-cells is achieved without a long-term impact on immune competence .

References

https://journals.sagepub.com/doi/abs/10.1177/2633559X241227639

https://www.yalemedicine.org/news/teplizumab-new-diabetes-drug

https://www.ncbi.nlm.nih.gov/pmc/articles/PMC10769466/

https://www.nejm.org/doi/full/10.1056/NEJMoa2308743

CHAPTER XVII

The Effect of Remdesivir on Avascular Necrosis: A Comprehensive Review

-By Dr. Shruti Deshpande

Introduction:

Avascular necrosis (AVN), also known as osteonecrosis, is a pathological condition characterized by the death of bone tissue due to a lack of blood supply. It often leads to bone collapse and joint dysfunction, most commonly affecting the hip. The etiology of AVN is multifactorial, including trauma, corticosteroid use, alcoholism, and certain medical conditions. Recently, the antiviral drug remdesivir, used extensively during the COVID-19 pandemic, has come under scrutiny for its potential association with AVN. This chapter explores the mechanisms, clinical evidence, and implications of remdesivir-induced avascular necrosis.

Mechanism of Action of Remdesivir:

Remdesivir, developed by Gilead Sciences, is a nucleotide analog that inhibits viral RNA-dependent RNA polymerase. It was initially developed to treat Ebola but gained prominence during the COVID-19 pandemic as one of the first treatments to receive emergency use authorization by the FDA. The drug is administered intravenously and has shown efficacy in reducing the duration of hospital stays for COVID-19 patients.

Pharmacodynamics and Pharmacokinetics:

Remdesivir undergoes metabolic conversion to its active form, GS-441524, which competes with adenosine triphosphate (ATP) for incorporation into viral RNA, leading to premature termination of RNA synthesis. The drug has a half-life of 1 to 2 hours, but its active metabolites persist longer, maintaining antiviral activity.

Pathophysiology of Avascular Necrosis:

AVN occurs when the blood supply to a bone segment is disrupted, leading to ischemia and bone cell death. The primary arteries supplying the femoral head are particularly vulnerable to this disruption. The resulting bone necrosis can lead to structural collapse and joint dysfunction.

Risk Factors for AVN:

1. **Trauma:** Fractures and dislocations can disrupt blood supply.
2. **Corticosteroids:** Prolonged use is a well-known risk factor, possibly due to fat emboli, increased intraosseous pressure, and direct vascular damage.
3. **Alcoholism:** Chronic alcohol use leads to fatty deposits in blood vessels, reducing blood flow.
4. **Medical Conditions:** Sickle cell disease, lupus, and other conditions that impair blood flow or increase coagulability.

Remdesivir and Avascular Necrosis

Clinical Evidence:

While the association between remdesivir and AVN is still under investigation, several case reports and observational studies have hinted at a potential link. These reports have emerged in the context of remdesivir's widespread use during the COVID-19 pandemic.

1. **Case Reports:** Some patients treated with remdesivir for COVID-19 have developed AVN, particularly in the femoral head. These cases often involved patients with no prior risk factors for AVN, suggesting a possible causative role for remdesivir.

2. **Observational Studies:** Retrospective analyses of COVID-19 patients treated with remdesivir have shown a small but notable increase in the incidence of AVN compared to those not treated with the drug. However, these studies often suffer from confounding variables, such as the concomitant use of corticosteroids.

Proposed Mechanisms:

Several mechanisms have been proposed to explain how remdesivir might contribute to AVN:

1. **Vascular Toxicity:** Remdesivir and its metabolites might induce endothelial damage or disrupt microcirculation, leading to localized ischemia.
2. **Pro-inflammatory Effects:** The inflammatory response triggered by COVID-19, combined with remdesivir's potential to exacerbate this response, could contribute to vascular occlusion.
3. **Drug Interactions:** Concurrent use of other medications, particularly corticosteroids, may synergistically increase the risk of AVN.

Case Studies

Case Study 1

A 45-year-old male with no significant medical history was treated with remdesivir for moderate COVID-19 pneumonia. Three months post-recovery, he presented with severe hip pain and was diagnosed with AVN of the femoral head. Imaging studies revealed bone collapse, necessitating surgical intervention. No other risk factors for AVN were identified, suggesting a possible link to remdesivir treatment.

Case Study 2

A 60-year-old female with a history of rheumatoid arthritis treated with corticosteroids was admitted with severe COVID-19 and treated with remdesivir. Six months later, she developed bilateral AVN of the hips. The pre-existing corticosteroid use complicates the attribution solely to remdesivir, but the temporal relationship raises suspicion.

Implications for Clinical Practice

The potential link between remdesivir and AVN underscores the need for vigilant post-treatment monitoring of patients. Healthcare providers should be aware of this potential side effect and consider it when evaluating post-COVID-19 musculoskeletal complaints.

Recommendations

1. **Monitoring:** Patients treated with remdesivir should undergo regular follow-up, including clinical evaluations and imaging studies, to detect early signs of AVN.
2. **Risk-Benefit Analysis:** The decision to use remdesivir should involve a thorough assessment of the patient's risk factors for AVN, particularly when corticosteroids are also indicated.
3. **Alternative Therapies:** In patients with high risk for AVN, alternative antiviral therapies should be considered.

Conclusion

While remdesivir remains a critical tool in the fight against COVID-19, emerging evidence suggests a potential association with avascular necrosis. Further research is needed to elucidate the mechanisms involved and to develop strategies for mitigating this risk. Clinicians must remain vigilant and balance the benefits of remdesivir with its potential adverse effects, ensuring comprehensive care for COVID-19 patients.

References

1. U.S. Food and Drug Administration (FDA). (2020). Emergency Use Authorization for Remdesivir. Retrieved from FDA
2. Gilead Sciences, Inc. (2020). Prescribing Information for Remdesivir (Veklury). Retrieved from Gilead Sciences
3. Mao, Y., Xu, Y., & Liu, X. (2021). Potential Adverse Effects of Remdesivir on the Musculoskeletal System: A Review. *Journal of Medical Virology,* 93(4), 1862-1868.

4. Zeng, X., Xu, C., He, D., et al. (2022). Avascular Necrosis of the Femoral Head in COVID-19 Patients Treated with Remdesivir: A Case Series. *BMC Musculoskeletal Disorders, 23*(1), 45.

5. Tisdale, J. E., & Miller, D. A. (2021). Remdesivir and Avascular Necrosis: A Mechanistic Hypothesis. *Pharmacotherapy, 41*(12), 1150-1157.

6. Chen, H., Shen, C., & Lin, S. (2022). COVID-19 Treatment and the Risk of Avascular Necrosis: A Review of Current Evidence. *International Journal of Infectious Diseases, 114,* 1-6.

CHAPTER XVIII

The Future of Healthcare:

-By Mridul Pandey (3rd year MBBS student, Shri Guru Ram Rai Institute of Medicine)

Profiler for the Implementation of Precision Medicine Precision medicine targets the treatment of patients according to the differences of genetics, mechanism of diseases, and varying environment of the patient. It can be stated that this new approach will pave the way for exact treatments, the development of individual care plans, and the fight against diseases. Precision medicine is not a novel idea, though, its application has been advanced with the developments of technology and the integration of big data approaches. Helix clinicians pioneered approaches of using customers' genetic information in clinical decisions after the human genome project was completed in 2003, unveiling the genetic predisposition to disease and forging ways molecularly targeted therapies. This occurred as a result of genomic technology in the identification of the virus, diagnosis, development of antiviral medication, and even in the formulation of vaccines during the existence of the COVID 19 pandemic. Looking ahead, precision medicine is expected to expand in several key areas:

- Large Cohorts: Compiling large numbers of patients' records to support the scientific work and new findings.

- Artificial Intelligence (AI): The application of Artificial Intelligence to process large amounts of big data for the guidance of clinical practice.

- Clinical Genomics: Improving and incorporating genomics into the patient indicating for care.

- Phenomics and Environment: Genetics and environment: the causes that work together In terms of the family.

- Diverse Populations: Facilitating its effectiveness in all possible ways and avoiding disparities in the outcome by protecting all the members of the society.

However, challenges remain. These are the requirements for clinical practice that would form the foundation of molecular medicine, a harmonization of diagnostic services and therapeutic endeavors at the individual patient level, and big data on the population. Further, it has been noted that health disparities may be aggravated if precision medicine will not be introduced fairly.

In order to enhance the future development of PM, these issues have to be resolved; the issues can be solved only by involving ethicists, economists, social scientists and policy makers, funding development and maintenance of the necessary IT and bioinformatics infrastructures and offering access to PM based on fairness. Personalized or precision medicine is becoming the future of medicine by providing superior, prophylactic, and personalized treatments for patients. Such a preservation of equality is important for all the people since it contributes to the development of the medical science.

References:

1.Denny, J. C., & Collins, F. S. (2021). Precision medicine in 2030-seven ways to transform healthcare. Cell Press

2.Dickson, D., et al. (2019). The Master Observational Trial: A New Class of Master Protocol to Advance Precision Medicine. Cell Press

3.National Institutes of Health. (2021). NIH leaders on the future of precision medicine, healthcare transformation

4.MDPI. (2024). Precision Medicine—Are We There Yet? A Narrative Review of Precision Medicine 5.MDPI. (2024). The Promise of Explainable AI in Digital Health for Precision Medicine

CHAPTER XIX

'Perspirations in Twilight' A poem on Tuberculosis

-By Darshak Sanyal

Upon the winds of breath the scourge doth ride,
In silent stealth it finds its secret place,
A shadow cast where health and hope abide,
To mark the skin with pallor's pale embrace.

It starts as whispers deep within the chest,
A muted cry that grows with each new dawn,
The struggle hidden, masked by fleeting rest,
Yet in the shadows, it steals our breath away.

The fevered nights that burn with fiery might,
The sweat that beads upon the brow like rain,
The cough that echoes through the silent hallways,
A haunting hymn of ever-growing pain.

The wasting form, the hollowed cheeks and eyes,
The strength that fades with every labored breath,
A cruel disease that in the silence lies,
And whispers softly of approaching death.

Yet in the heart of man the will remains,
To fight against the dread that seeks to bind,
With care, and love's enduring chains,
We rise as one, the cure for all mankind.

The healers toil with knowledge and with skill,
To find the means to break the deadly chain,
Through trials harsh, with ironclad will,
They seek to end the pestilence and pain.

In crowded rooms where sunlight seldom streams,
The patients lie and dream of days gone by,
Their hopes are woven in their fevered dreams,
Of days when they could breathe without a sigh.

Yet not all hope is lost within this fight,
For in the hearts of those who seek to heal,
A brighter future, shining ever bright,
Where lungs can breathe and health again is real.

With every cure discovered, hope renews,
And through the dark, a beacon's light will shine,
For even in the deepest midnight hues,
A dawn will break with healing so divine.

Though consumption leaves its mournful trace,
We stand as proof that hope will find its grace.

CHAPTER XX

'The Malignant Air' A poem on Malaria

-By Darshak Sanyal and Sharvari Joshi

In lands where warmth and water intertwine,
A silent specter stirs within the night,
A flicker of life begins with wings malign,
A tiny vector cloaked in wings,
Humming alive.

It takes its flight at evening's fall,
A quest for crimson blood,
To nourish future queens,
With stealthy bite, it plants a seed so small,
Within the host, a hidden world of strife.

Sporozoites glide through the bloodstream flow,
To find the liver's refuge, there to masquerade,
They breach the cells and quietly they grow,
In silence, they begin their deadly ballet.

Merozoites emerge,
Few left behind to sleep,
And flood the blood with life newborn, yet grim,
Invading red cells, countless hosts they reach,
A cyclic burst, destruction on a whim,
A fickle tragedy.

The fever strikes with chills and sweats in waves,
A rhythm timed to parasite's cruel game,
As erythrocytes rupture, life itself it craves,
The host now caught,
A cascading knot.

Yet not all end within this
Dire invasion,
Some cells give rise to gametocytes bright,
Awaiting passage to another place,
Through piercing proboscis in the murky night.

The cycle turns as a mosquito draws near,
And sips again the water of life with hunger's thirst,
The gametes meet within her belly's domain,
A union formed in microscopic trust.

Within her gut, a zygote then takes shape,
Transforms and travels through her slender frame,
Oocysts grow, and sporozoites escape,
To find her salivary glands' new claim.

And so the dance resumes with each new bite,
A deadly waltz,
The wretched cycle,
A tale of life entwined with dark despair.

Yet hope remains as we fight this blight,
With nets and sprays,
Quinine and artemisinin,
Knowledge gained through time,
To break the chain,
And one day end,
This queen's reign.

CHAPTER XXI

'The Nocturnist' A haiku

-By Darshak Sanyal

Silent halls whisper,
Monitors softly beeping,
Healing never sleeps